Jermaine Collier Jr:NASM-CPT, USATF COACH

FIT FAMILY BLUEPRINT

A BUSY PARENT'S GUIDE TO HEALTH, HAPPINESS, AND HOME WORKOUTS

Copyright © 2024 by Jermaine Collier Jr.

All rights reserved. No part of this publication may be reproduced, distributed, or transmitted in any form or by any means, including photocopying, recording, or other electronic or mechanical methods, without the prior written permission of the publisher, except in the case of brief quotations embodied in critical reviews and certain other noncommercial uses permitted by copyright law.

First Edition

ISBN 9798345540114

Published by Team JMC LLC
Cambridge, MA

This book is a work of nonfiction. All efforts have been made to ensure accuracy; however, the publisher does not assume responsibility for any loss or injury resulting from the use of this book. Consult a qualified health professional before beginning any exercise program or nutritional changes.

For permissions, contact:
jmcfitness@jmcfitness.net

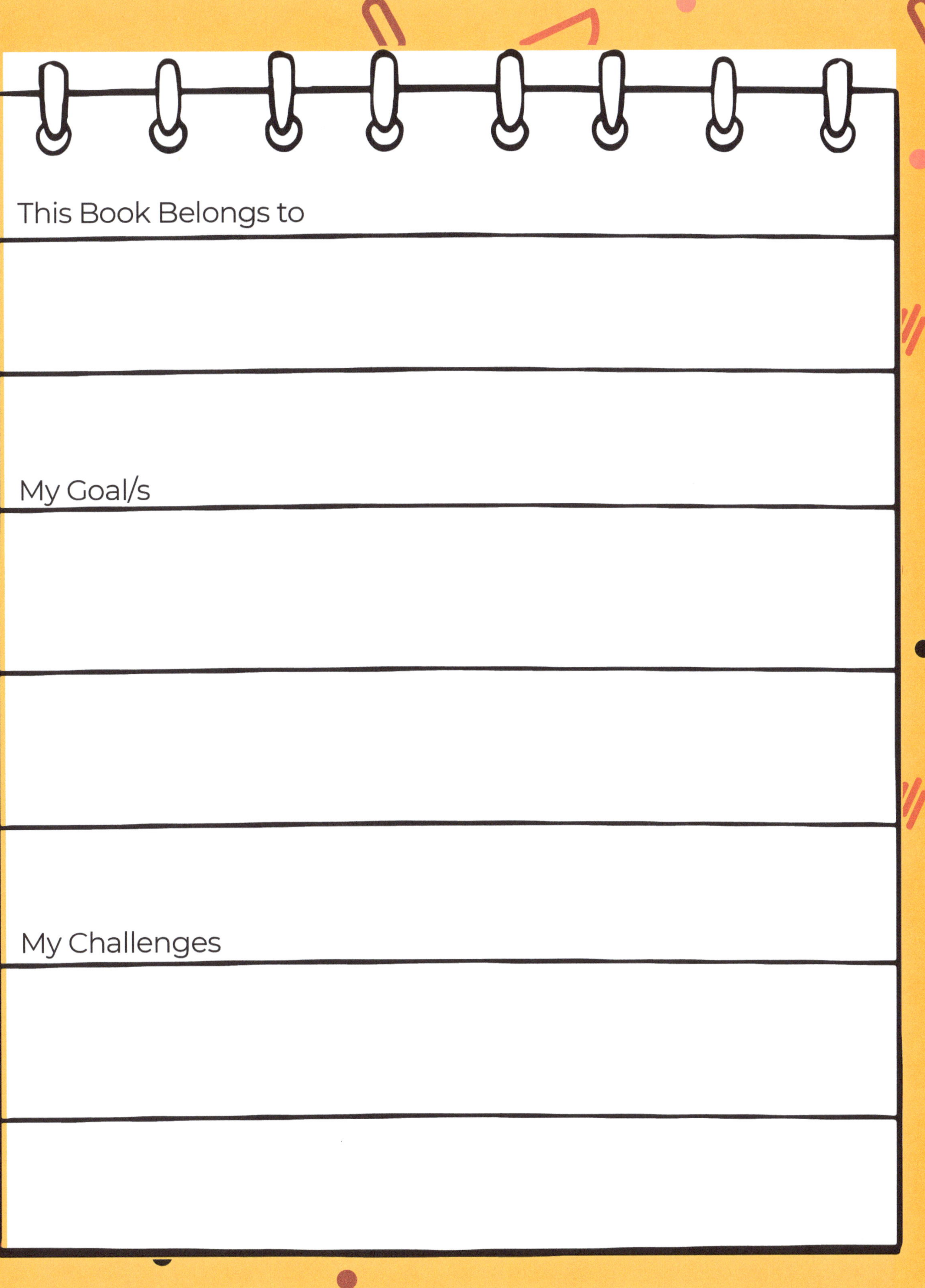

This Book Belongs to
My Goal/s
My Challenges

Table of Contents
Purpose of the Ebook

Introduction

Purpose of the Ebook

This guide is designed for busy parents who want to improve their health, lose weight, tone up, or build muscle without having to go to a gym or buy costly equipment. It offers practical fitness routines you can do at home, with or without your kids, and includes essential nutrition tips for families aiming to live healthier lives. You'll find everything you need to make fitness a part of your family's routine.

A Personal Story: Childhood Athlete to Fit Parent

Fitness has always been part of my life. Growing up, I was inspired by my dad, he was always active playing basketball and football, and my mom, who participated in High school track and field. My journey began when I turned eight. I wanted to play football, my parents agreed but decided I'd need to balance it with track. I enjoyed participating in both sports. However, at 11 years old I wanted to quit due to the mental and physical demands of being a multi-sport student athlete. My parents quickly educated me that giving up is the only way to truly lose, also that they didn't raise me to be a quitter. By 13 years old, I was already learning the value of hard work, discipline, and commitment. It was challenging, but a few wins under my belt made it worth it.

As I grew, track and field became a serious focus. I followed in my mom's footsteps, competing in hurdles & sprints. I was fortunate to be coached by Alfonso Jennings who was like a second father. Coach Jennings taught me that anything worth having doesn't come easy. He prepared me both mentally and physically for the challenges of the sport. There were still times I wanted to quit, but my parents reminded me how far I'd come, motivating me to stay committed. By my senior year, all the hard work had paid off—I earned county, state, and national champion titles, earning a full athletic scholarship to a top D1 school.

In college, I gained interest in my family's health history. Through curiosity, I noticed how some lifestyle choices benefited my journey & others did not. After witnessing loved ones and others who struggled with health issues, I began to understand the value of living a healthy lifestyle.

I realized that fitness was more than a routine—it was a path to longevity and a way to break generational health patterns. I made a promise to my mom and myself to stay committed to fitness, not just for my own well-being but to set an example for my family.

When I became a father, balancing family, work, and fitness brought new challenges. My wife, who was also an accomplished track athlete faced a complicated pregnancy. Our first child had some early health concerns, which shifted my focus entirely to supporting my family. Fitness had always been part of my identity, and I started to feel the loss. Long workdays made fitness feel impossible, and soon I felt the absence of that physical and mental outlet. I was often exhausted due to lack of sleep, on top of more responsibilities & priorities. I knew the journey would be tough to start and commit to. Understanding the journey ahead, I had no motivation to start until one day of quality father & son time.

While my wife was out, my son was wide awake during "nap time." Trying to keep him entertained, I picked him up and started doing body squats as a form of lulling. To my surprise, he began to laugh and didn't appreciate the breaks in between sets. His pure enjoyment was motivating! Through the experience I realized that I could blend fitness and family time. From that moment, I began creating simple home workouts that my wife and I could do together, even with the kids around. As we saw results and our energy increased, fitness became part of our family routine. And just as we built momentum, we got news that we were expecting our second child. This time, we had a strategy to keep fitness as a part of our lives, no matter what.

Today, fitness is woven into our family life. We enjoy spending active, quality time together, and our kids see exercise as fun. My journey has shown me that fitness isn't just about physical strength—it's about building resilience, creating memories, and setting an example. Our family now has a foundation of health, and it's something I'm proud to pass on to my children every day.

A Note from My Wife

"My fitness journey has had ups and downs, but it's been worth every step. After our pregnancies, particularly with the complications I faced, fitness helped me heal from the inside out. It was essential in regaining my strength and confidence, and I'm more secure now than ever. This shift has positively impacted our kids. They're growing up seeing health as a priority, in a household where their parents love what they do. Our two sons see a healthy, happy father as their role model, which is something I'm grateful for every day."

Chapter 1:
The Parent Fitness Challenge

Understanding the Challenge

As parents, finding time, energy, and resources for fitness can be daunting. But even brief, consistent sessions can bring lasting changes. Fitness doesn't require hours in the gym. It can be achieved in small steps by fitting it into your busy life with kids, work, and home responsibilities.

Step 1: Setting Simple, Realistic Goals

Start with goals that feel achievable and rewarding:

- Weight Loss: Aim for steady progress by incorporating daily movement and mindful eating.
- Toning Up: Focus on short, effective strength exercises you can do anywhere, requiring minimal time or equipment.
- Consistency: Set up a schedule of 10–30-minute routines designed to fit into your family's daily rhythm.

Example Goal: "Lose 5 pounds over the next month by adding 15–20 minutes of daily movement and making one mindful change to each meal."

- Incorporate Daily Movement: Try to walk for 10 minutes after meals or do a quick family dance session after dinner. These small, regular bursts of movement add up and help burn calories.

Mindful Eating Tips:

- Swap soda or sugary drinks for water (Juice fruits for flavor).
- Add a vegetable to every meal.
- Practice portion control by serving meals on smaller plates.

By focusing on small, sustainable changes, you'll see steady progress without overwhelming your schedule.

Remember, progress builds over time, and every small step counts.

Chapter 2:
Building a Fit Mindset

Step 2: Accountability and Consistency

Accountability is essential to your fitness journey. Try tracking progress on a family chart (maybe on the fridge), involving your spouse or kids as workout partners, or simply celebrating each milestones make fitness a priority. Weaving it into your routine instead of seeing it as a separate task makes a difference .

How It Works:

- Each day, everyone adds a checkmark or a sticker next to their goal when it's completed.
- At the end of each week, celebrate the family's progress! Try a special reward like a family movie night, choosing a favorite dinner, or a fun outdoor activity.
- Involving your spouse or kids keeps everyone engaged, motivated, and accountable.

Step 3: Self-Care and Positive Thinking

MINDSET MATTERS more than you might assume! Prioritizing sleep, self-care, and daily movement, no matter how small, can boost your motivation and consistency. View fitness as part of your identity and set an example for your family to adopt healthy habits for life.

How It Works:

- Prioritize Sleep & Self-Care: Set family "wind-down" time, turning off all screens (if possible) 30 minutes before bed to help everyone rest well.
- Add Daily Movement: Do a 5 minute morning stretch routine or a quick evening walk together to make fitness a regular, positive part of your day.
- Build a Healthy Family Identity: Use affirmations! example "Our family prioritizes our bodies and minds," to reinforce healthy habits.

Fit Tip: A fitness routine doesn't need to be long to be effective—small, consistent actions lead to lasting results.

Chapter 3:
Overcoming Challenges

Managing a Busy Schedule:
Making time for fitness as a parent can be tough, but even small moments of movement make a difference. Finding those pockets of time—early in the morning or after the kids are asleep can be a game-changer.
For example, in my journey, there were days when long work hours and family responsibilities made it feel impossible to prioritize fitness. But I learned to adapt by using short, effective workouts I could do at home.

Breaking Through Plateaus *(State of Little/no change)***:**
Progress isn't always linear (almost never). Hitting a plateau can feel frustrating, but small changes can revive your motivation and keep you pushing forward. Introducing a new activity, changing your routine, or words of encouragement can make a world of difference. For me, plateau moments became opportunities to adapt. During my high school years in track, I wanted to quit on a few occasions because of the intense demands, but with the encouragement of my coach, family, & positive self talk, I was able to push through by changing up my routines and challenging myself in new ways.

Handling Setbacks:
Missing workouts or taking a few days off is natural, especially with a busy schedule. Consistency is what's most important, not perfection. Fitness isn't about being perfect; it's about building a lifestyle over time. Every step, no matter how small, is progress toward a healthier family. When my wife and I first became parents, there were many times when fitness took a back seat, especially during her recovery. It was common to feel like we weren't doing "enough," but we kept resorting to small, consistent actions (daily walk & talks). Little by little, we built our momentum and made fitness a fun, family focused part of our day.

Chapter 4:
Family-Friendly Home Workouts

Family workouts can be simple, adaptable, and engaging for different fitness levels. Each circuit is designed to take 20–30 minutes, can be done with or without kids, and focuses on functional strength and endurance. Aim for two or three rounds of each circuit 3 day out of the week (include at least 1 rest day in between completed circuits).

Warm-Up (5 Minutes/1 minute each exercise)
- March in Place
- Jumping Jacks
- Bodyweight Squats
- Arm Circles
- High Knees

Workout Circuits
1. **Strength Circuit**
   - Squats: 12 reps (hold your child or a weighted item)
   - Push-Ups: 10–15 reps (on knees for beginners, full for advanced)
   - Bent Over Rows: 12 reps (use a filled bag or child's weight for resistance)
   - Glute Bridges: 15 reps (add weight on hips for resistance)
2. **Cardio & Core Circuit**
   - Mountain Climbers: 30 seconds
   - Plank with Shoulder Taps: 10 per side
   - Lunges with a Twist: 10 per side (holding weight or child)
   - Toe Touches: 15 reps

Five minute cooldown stretch

- Toe Touch (1 minute)
- Side Stretch (30 seconds each side)
- ad Stretch (30 seconds each leg)
- Shoulder Stretch (30 seconds each arm)
- Child's Pose (1 minute)

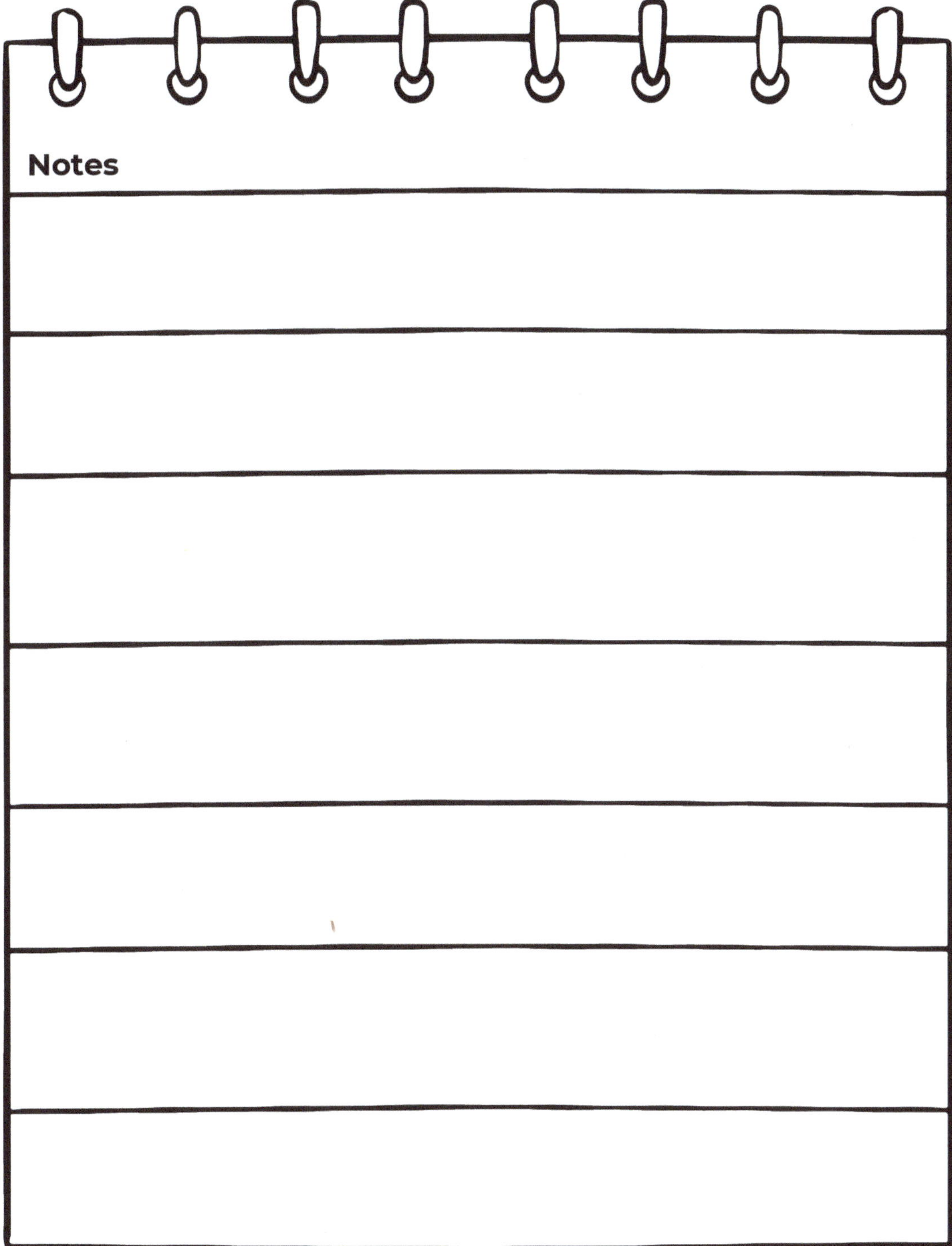

Notes

Chapter 5:
Nutrition Guide for Busy Families

Balanced Family Eating Nutrition is essential for energy, focus, and achieving fitness goals. Here's a simple, nutritious guide for family-friendly meals that support weight loss and toning.

Quick Meal Guide

1. **Breakfast Options**
   - Greek yogurt with berries and granola
   - Whole-grain toast with almond butter and banana slices
   - Smoothie with spinach, banana, protein powder, and almond milk
2. **Lunch Ideas**
   - Wrap with lean protein (turkey, chicken), veggies, and hummus
   - Quinoa bowl with vegetables, a drizzle of olive oil, and protein
   - Chickpea and mixed greens salad with cherry tomatoes
3. **Dinner Choices**
   - Chicken or tofu stir-fry with mixed veggies and brown rice
   - Sheet pan salmon with roasted sweet potatoes and asparagus
   - Spaghetti squash with marinara and ground turkey
4. **Snacks**
   - Apple slices with peanut butter
   - Veggie sticks with hummus
   - Cottage cheese with pineapple

Hydration: Aim for 8+ glasses of water daily, and limit sugary drinks.

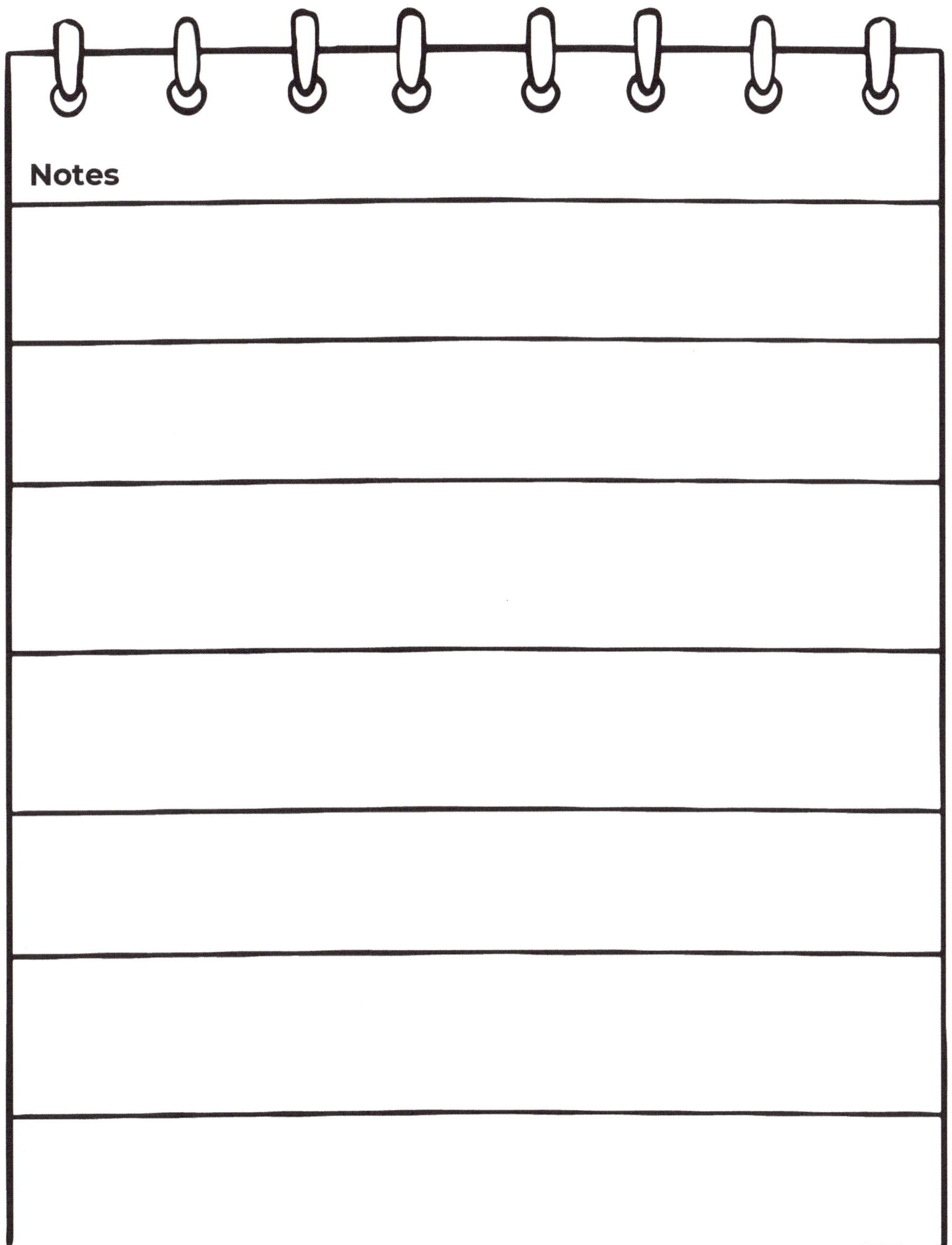

Notes

Chapter 6:
Staying Motivated & Involving the Family

Making Fitness Fun for Everyone Family workouts are a great opportunity to bond with one another. When kids see fitness as play, they're more likely to make it a habit. Enjoy active family time, from weekend hikes to dance offs.

Weekly Challenges Keep fitness fresh and fun:

- *Step Challenge:* Track family steps and aim for a weekly goal.
- *Healthy Recipe of the Week:* Try one new nutritious recipe together.
- *Outdoor Fun:* Plan an active outing each weekend, like a hike, family tag, or family game.
- *Indoor Fun:* Plan an indoor activity each weekend, like a family circuit or family game.

Outdoor Activity: *Roll & Move Family Fitness Dice Game*
This outdoor version of the dice game incorporates more space for active, whole-body movements. Get ready for a fun family workout with plenty of room to move! Modify exercises to accommodate fitness levels.

Dice Setup

- Die 1 (Duration/Reps): One die with the following options:
    - Side 1: "30 seconds"
    - Side 2: "45 seconds"
    - Side 3: "60 seconds"
    - Side 4: "10 reps"
    - Side 5: "15 reps"
    - Side 6: "20 reps"

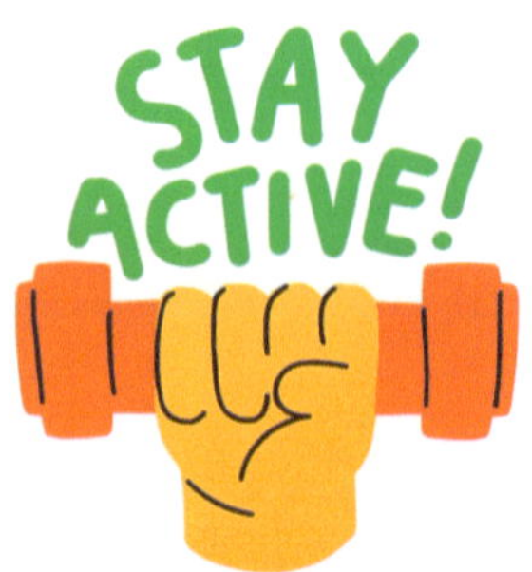

- Die 2 (Exercise): Another die with the following exercises:
  - Side 1: Walking Lunges (Lower Body)
  - Side 2: Squat Jumps (Lower Body)
  - Side 3: Push-Ups (Upper Body)
  - Side 4: Shoulder Taps (Upper Body)
  - Side 5: Bear Crawl (Full Body)
  - Side 6: Jumping Jacks (Full Body)

How to Play

1. Roll the Dice: One player rolls both dice to determine the activity. The first die decides the duration (time/reps) and whether it includes running, while the second die determines the exercise.
2. Complete the Exercise: Everyone does the chosen exercise for the rolled time or reps. For example, if the roll is "30 seconds" and "Bear Crawl," the family performs a bear crawl for 30 seconds.
3. Move Around the Yard/Playground: Use your outdoor space by designating areas for each exercise. For instance:
   - Lunges or Squat Jumps can be done in one spot,
   - Running laps can be a jog around the yard,
   - Bear Crawls or Jumping Jacks can be done in open spaces.
4. Take Turns: Rotate who rolls the dice, allowing each person to "lead" the family for one roll. Continue for as many rounds as you'd like!

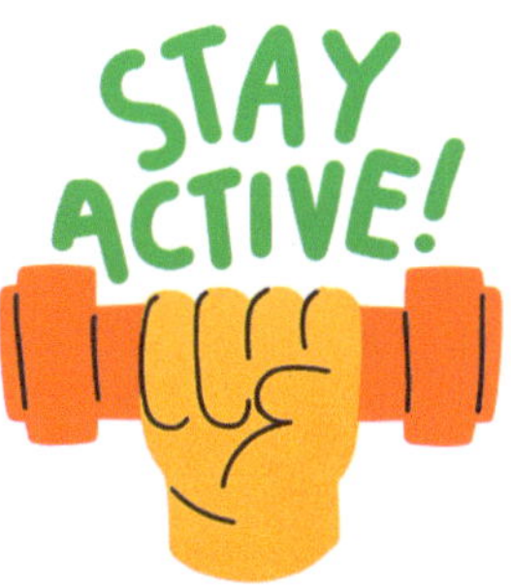

Indoor Activity: *Roll & Move Family Fitness Dice Game*
In this game, you'll use two dice to determine the exercise and
the duration/reps. This makes the workout unpredictable and
fun, while allowing everyone to go at their own pace! Modify
exercises to accommodate fitness levels.
Dice Setup
- Die 1 (Duration/Reps): One die with the following options:
    - Side 1: "30 seconds"
    - Side 2: "45 seconds"
    - Side 3: "60 seconds"
    - Side 4: "10 reps"
    - Side 5: "15 reps"
    - Side 6: "20 reps"
- Die 2 (Exercise): Another die with the following exercises:
    - Side 1: Squats (Lower Body)
    - Side 2: Lunges (Lower Body)
    - Side 3: Push-Ups (Upper Body)
    - Side 4: Shoulder Taps (Upper Body)
    - Side 5: Jumping Jacks (Full Body)
    - Side 6: Mountain Climbers (Full Body)

How to Play

1. Roll the Dice: One player rolls both dice. The first die
   determines the duration or reps, and the second die
   determines the exercise.
2. Complete the Exercise: Everyone does the chosen exercise
   for the rolled time or reps. For example, if you roll "15 reps"
   on Die 1 and "Squats" on Die 2, everyone does 15 squats.
3. Take Turns: After each turn, another player rolls the dice to
   set the next exercise and duration/reps. Continue for as
   many rounds as you like.

Optional Variations

- Power Round: Once every 5 rolls, double the reps or add 15 seconds to the time for a fun challenge.
- Family Relay: Pair up and take turns within teams, so one team rests while the other completes their roll.

This game keeps everyone moving, adds a playful element of chance, and allows each family member to adjust their intensity as needed. Play some upbeat music and enjoy the fun fitness routine together!

Tracking Progress Together Use a family chart or app to log workouts, set milestones, and celebrate accomplishments. Each win is a reason to celebrate!

Scan the QR Code to Order

- 4 Dice Set: Keep workouts varied and enjoyable with exercise, duration, and rep options that work for all levels!
- Dry-Erase Board: Track your family's scores, set goals, and celebrate wins together. This reusable board helps make fitness a lasting habit.

Conclusion & Next Steps

Celebrate Your Success Congratulations on taking the first steps toward a healthier family life! Remember, no mater how small, every action counts! Every activity brings you closer to long term health and wellness. Celebrate the progress you've made and know that this is just the beginning of a beneficial lifestyle shift.

Stay Connected with Our Community To keep the momentum going, join our online community (Instagram, & Facebook group) where you can find support, share your journey, and connect with other parents who are on a similar journey. Being part of a community is an effective way to stay motivated and keep learning.

Exclusive Resources & Tips Follow us on social media for weekly tips, new workouts, and exclusive resources to help you and your family stay active and healthy. By staying connected, you'll receive advice, motivational content, and family friendly health tips as a thank you for joining us on this journey.

Take the Next Step with JMC Fitness Ready for the next step? JMC Fitness offers personalized online training and coaching tailored for busy parents who want to continue building their health and fitness journey. From customized plans to one-on-one support, our goal is to make fitness work for your life. Visit our website for more details, or contact us directly for a free consultation.

Keep Going—For Yourself and Your Family Remember, the journey to fitness is ongoing. With each step, you're building a legacy of health, wellness, and active living for your family. Continue to embrace each moment, enjoy the quality time, and know that every effort you make is bringing you closer to a healthier, happier life together.

Leave a Review & Share Your Journey

We'd be happy to Hear From You! Your feedback helps us make each resource that much better for other parents who are on the path to a healthier family life. If you found this guide helpful, we'd love for you to leave a review. Your experience can inspire others to start their journey too!

How to Leave a Review

- Scan the QR Code: Simply scan the QR code below to be taken directly to the review page.
- Share Your Experience: Tell us how this guide has helped you, what you enjoyed most, and any ideas you have for future resources.
- Submit Your Review: Once submitted, your review will help other parents discover this guide and begin their own fitness journey.

Share Your Progress on Social Media!
Tag us on instagram (@teamjmcllc) to share a post, reel, or story of how using this guide has helped you. Witnessing your progress not only motivates others, but also reminds you and your family of the amazing steps you're taking. Also, we may share your story on our page as part of our supportive fitness community.

A Special Thank You!
Leave a review and send us a screenshot by email or direct message for a free bonus resource! We're grateful to have the opportunity to assist you on your journey and can't wait to see how far hit take you!

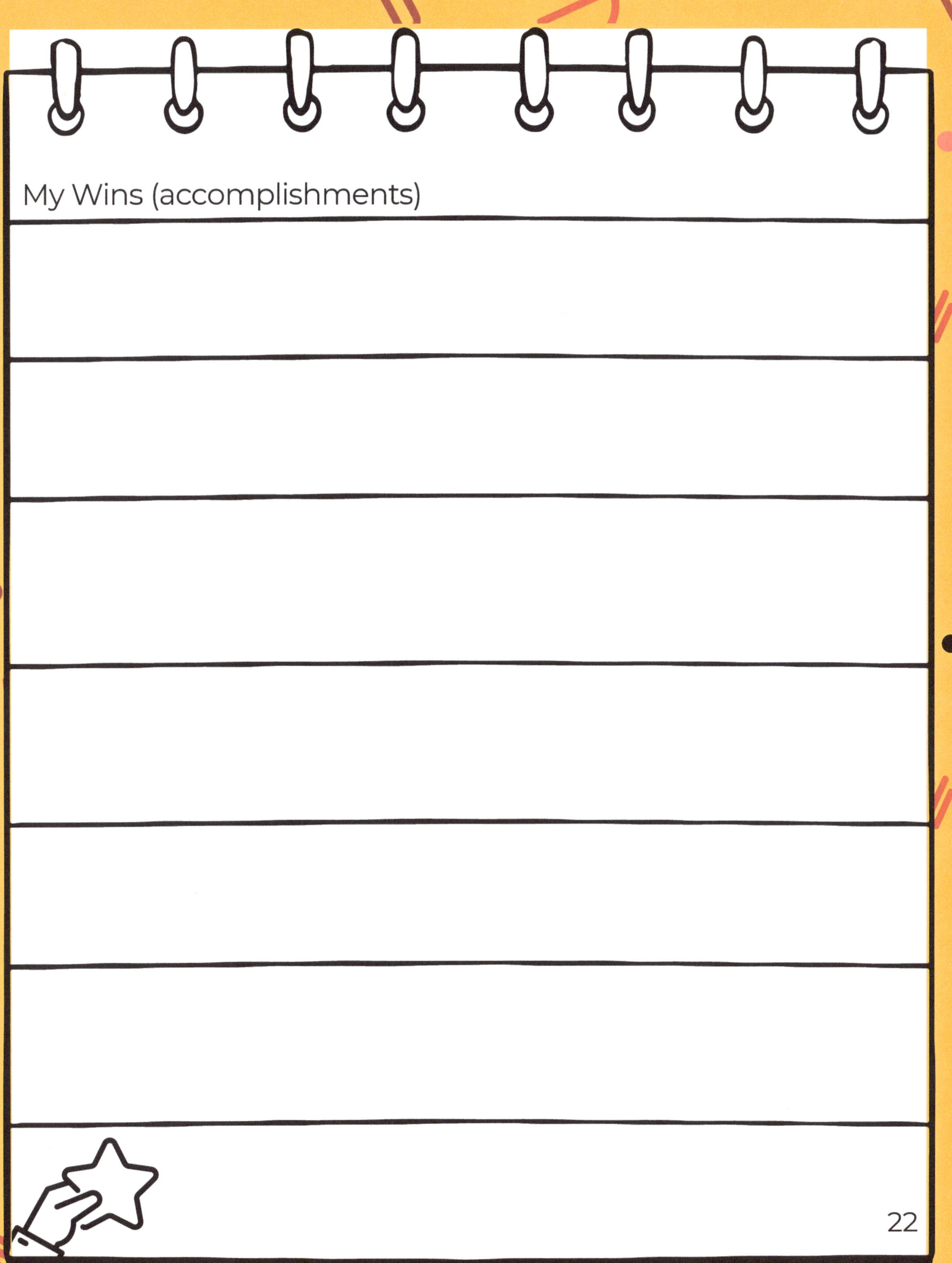

My Wins (accomplishments)

www.ingramcontent.com/pod-product-compliance
Lightning Source LLC
Chambersburg PA
CBHW040038240726

48664CB00003B/984